Problems with the Eyes and Seeing

Beyond the Basics

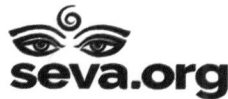

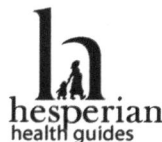

seva.org

hesperian
health guides

Oakland, California, USA

PROBLEMS WITH THE EYES AND SEEING CAN BE IMPROVED WITH YOUR HELP. If you are a health worker, community organizer, teacher, or anyone with ideas or suggestions for ways this booklet could be changed to better meet the needs of your community, please write to Hesperian. Thank you for your help.

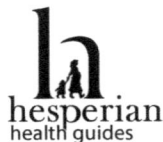

hesperian
health guides

2860 Telegraph Avenue
Oakland, California 94609, USA
hesperian@hesperian.org
www.hesperian.org

Contents

Problems with the Eyes and Seeing

Basic Care for Eyes

Keeping the face and the area around the eyes clean and protected from too much sun, wind, and injury will prevent many common problems that harm eyes or make them irritated, red, or painful. Eating nutritious food also prevents many eye problems.

Injuries can damage vision or cause blindness. Act quickly: go to the closest hospital or health clinic for a serious eye injury or for danger signs (see page 8). They can help you find an eye specialist if one is needed.

When far away or very close objects are difficult to see, the right kind of eyeglasses often helps people see much better. Because vision changes over time, you may need new eyeglasses every so often.

For adults, cataracts (page 19) and glaucoma (page 20) are common causes of vision loss that can lead to blindness. Treatment can help restore vision or stop it from getting worse. Knowing about the eye and its parts will help you keep the eyes healthy and take care of eye problems.

THE PARTS OF THE EYE

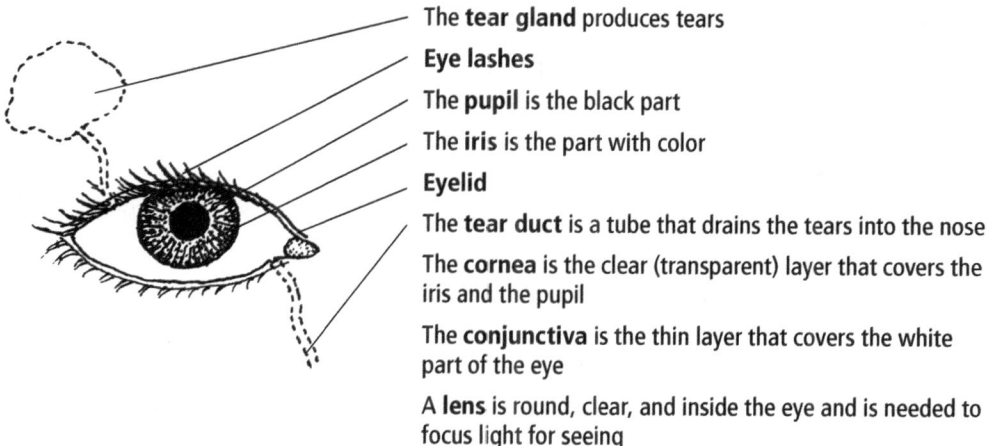

The **tear gland** produces tears

Eye lashes

The **pupil** is the black part

The **iris** is the part with color

Eyelid

The **tear duct** is a tube that drains the tears into the nose

The **cornea** is the clear (transparent) layer that covers the iris and the pupil

The **conjunctiva** is the thin layer that covers the white part of the eye

A **lens** is round, clear, and inside the eye and is needed to focus light for seeing

When eyes are healthy:

- The eyelids open and shut easily and the eye lashes curve outward, not in toward the eye.
- The white part is all white, smooth, and moist.
- The cornea, the clear covering of the iris and pupil, is shiny, smooth and transparent.
- The pupil is black and round. This black part reacts to more or less light by becoming smaller or bigger.

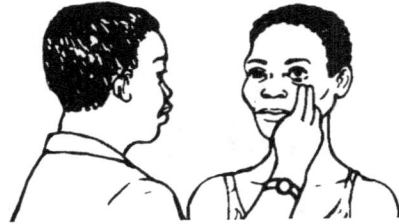

Keep the eyes clean

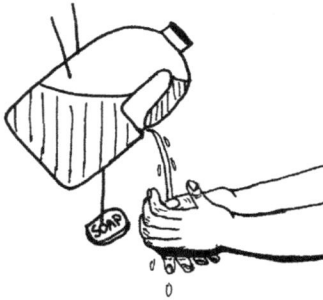

To help prevent many eye problems, wash your face often. This keeps dirt and germs from getting in the eye and causing problems.

You do not need a lot of water to wash the face. You can make a Tippy-Tap from a clean plastic bottle or container (see Water and Sanitation: Keys to Staying Healthy, page 4). Let the air dry your face and hands to avoid infections from sharing cloth or towels.

When eyes are infected, clean them often with a clean cloth and clean water. Wipe gently from the corner of the eye nearest to the nose outward to the corner of the eye by the ear. Use a different part of the cloth to clean each eye and then wash the cloth well and dry it before you use it again.

Wash your hands with soap before and after cleaning eyes that are infected to prevent spreading infection.

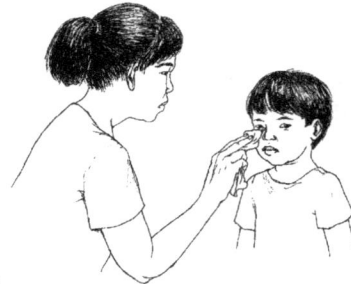

How to remove dirt or an eyelash from the eye

Have the person close her eyes and move her eyes around from side to side, and up and down. Then, while you hold her eyelid open, have her look up and down again. This makes the eye produce tears that often wash out the dirt. Another way of making tears is to gently rub the good eye. This produces tears in both eyes. Do not rub the sore eye.

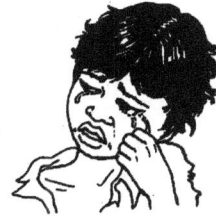

Something trapped under the eyelid can scratch or scrape your eye, so do not rub the eye. Tears can help wash it out.

Or you can try to remove the bit of dirt or eyelash with clean water. Use only clean water, not any other liquid. Hold the eye open while rinsing with water from a cup (or by gently squirting water with a clean syringe and no needle). The person can lie down or tilt her head back while you pour water so it runs from the inside (near the nose) to the outside of the eye (near the ear).

If you can see it, the bit of dirt can be gently removed with the corner of a damp, clean cloth, tissue, or cotton swab.

When dirt is under the upper eyelid, you may only be able to see it by turning the upper eyelid over a cotton swab. Ask the person to look down while you do this.

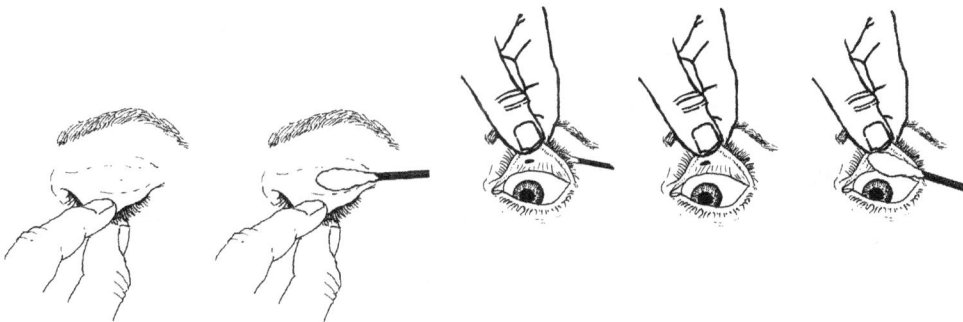

Remove the eyelash or bit of dirt with the corner of a clean cloth, tissue, or cotton swab. Always move the dirt away from the eye.

If you cannot get the dirt out easily, put a small amount of antibiotic eye ointment where the irritation is felt, protect the eye (see page 12), and send the person for medical help.

Workplace dangers, pollution, and sun harm eyes

Chemicals, air and water pollution, and the strong rays in sunlight (called ultraviolet or UV rays) can irritate the eyes and cause problems. At home or at work, eyes can be injured by many things, or burned by chemicals.

- **Cooking:** smoke from cooking fires and stoves irritates and dries the eyes. This affects women and children most.
- **Air pollution:** dust and chemicals in the air affect the eyes of everyone who works or plays outside, especially children.
- **Water pollution:** chemicals from factories or mines, pesticides, and sewage are released into rivers or lakes, irritating the eyes and skin of people who bathe or wash clothes there.
- **Agriculture:** tools, dirt, rocks, tree branches, poisonous plants, chemical fertilizers and pesticides can all damage the eyes.
- **Outside:** sun, dust, and wind can irritate the eyes.
- **Riding a motorcycle** without protecting eyes can lead to eye injury.
- **Chemicals:** factory workers, farmers, miners, janitors, domestic workers and others use chemicals. If chemicals touch the eye, they can burn it very quickly (page 11).
- **Machines or equipment:** pieces of metal or wood can break off and injure the eye, as can high heat, sparks, or flames.
- **Office and factory workers:** having to focus the eyes on one task for many hours strains the eyes.

Safety glasses and goggles protect eyes from injury

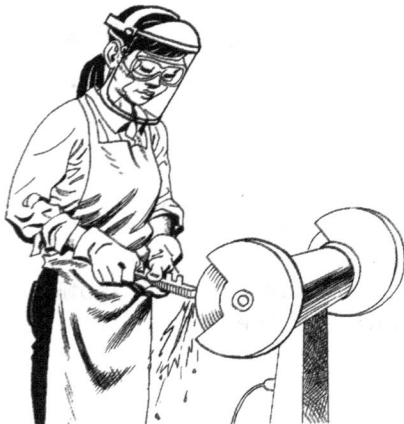

All glasses help protect eyes. Use safety glasses or safety goggles when using machines or power tools, riding a motorcycle, or if you are working with pesticides or other chemicals.

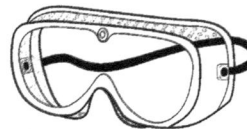

For more on protecting eyes in the workplace, see Hesperian's *Workers' Guide to Health and Safety*.

Hats and sunglasses protect eyes from sun

People outside in strong sunlight can protect their eyes by wearing a hat and, if possible, dark glasses. Glasses that are made to screen out UV (ultraviolet) sun rays are best. Protection from the sun may slow the advance of some types of cataracts (see page 19). Even after many years of too much sun, using hats and sunglasses may prevent eye problems from getting worse.

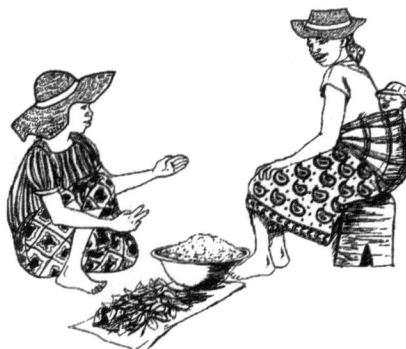

Avoid eye strain

Working where there is not enough light, looking at the screen of your computer or mobile phone all the time, or focusing your eyes for many hours on something close is hard on the eyes. Reduce eye strain by improving lighting and regularly looking away at something across the room. Older workers may need reading glasses for close-up work (page 29).

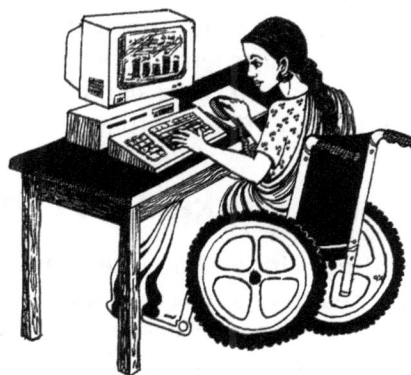

First look at something close to you.

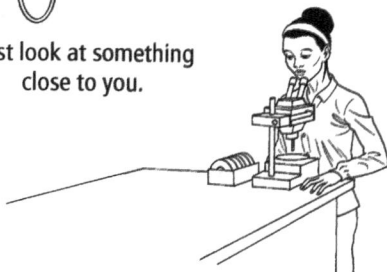

Then look away to something about 3 to 4 meters away for 20 seconds.

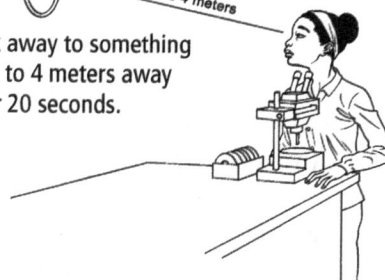

3 to 4 meters

Do this a few times each hour. Also, it helps to move your eyes around: keep your head still and move your eyes to look up one wall, around the ceiling, and down the other wall.

Care for the eyes with good food

Many foods that help the body stay healthy also help people have good vision. Foods especially good for eye health include:

- Vegetables: leafy greens, pepper, peas, beans, sweet potato, carrot, and pumpkin
- Fruits: mango, papaya, orange, and avocado
- Fish, nuts, and whole grains

Eating nutritious foods during pregnancy helps the developing baby's eyes. Breastfeeding babies and making sure young children eat green and orange vegetables and fruits can prevent vitamin A deficiency (page 23).

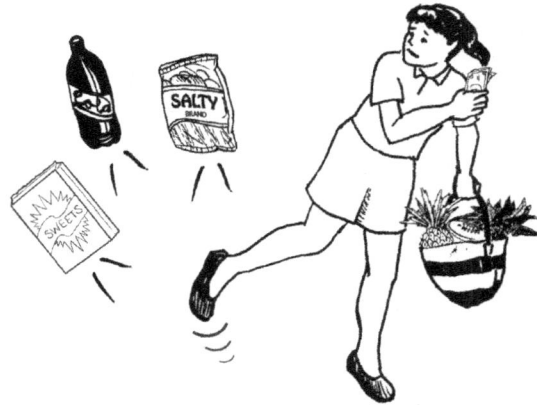

Save your money for nutritious foods and keep away the salt and sugar.

Health workers and community eye health

Dealing with eye emergencies is unfortunately common for health workers and health promoters, but everyday eye and vision problems may not be. When health workers learn to recognize early signs of eye problems, they can help people improve their vision and prevent people from losing their sight.

- Learn to look for redness, swelling, itching, or gray spots in the eyes when you see patients – and what each sign means and how to treat it.
- Make it easier for women to receive eye exams and eye treatment. Their work and family roles make them more likely to suffer eye problems.
- Help people know what home remedies and commercial products might be dangerous for the eye and not to spend money on false cures.
- Organize a yearly vision check for children at school and train teachers to recognize signs of eye problems, especially poor vision.
- Refer older people for treatment if they have cataracts.
- Help people over the age of 40 get reading glasses if they need them.
- Make your community a safe place for people who are blind (page 30).

Health workers can also share information on programs and eye hospitals that offer low-cost or free care for eye problems and emergencies. Organize community members to get vision testing, eyeglasses, and cataract surgery at not-for-profit and government organized events (see page 20).

Common eye problems by age:

Babies' eye infections need to be treated. Some of these are prevented by cleaning the baby's eyes and using eye ointment at birth (see page 33).

Young children's vision problems may be hard to notice. Starting at 6 months old, see if the child's eyes move and follow a light or a toy when you move it around. A child with a wandering or crossed eye can be helped (page 24) and glasses may help with poor vision. For children with very limited or no vision, Hesperian's book *Helping Children Who Are Blind* shows many ways to help a blind child develop her skills.

School-age children who cannot see clearly cannot tell you they need eyeglasses because they do not know what good vision would be like. A child who has headaches, squints a lot or is having difficulty in school or playing games may have a vision problem and need eyeglasses. It is also a good idea to learn what to do if there is an eye injury from sports or fighting at school.

Any child can get eye injuries. Keep chemicals and sharp objects locked away and out of reach of children.

Adult vision may change at any age and sometimes eyeglasses can help. If a person has diabetes or high blood pressure, treatment to manage these problems will help prevent further harm to the eyes. Different kinds of work make some eye injuries or eye conditions more likely (page 4).

Older adults are more likely to develop cataracts (page 19) and need reading glasses (page 29).

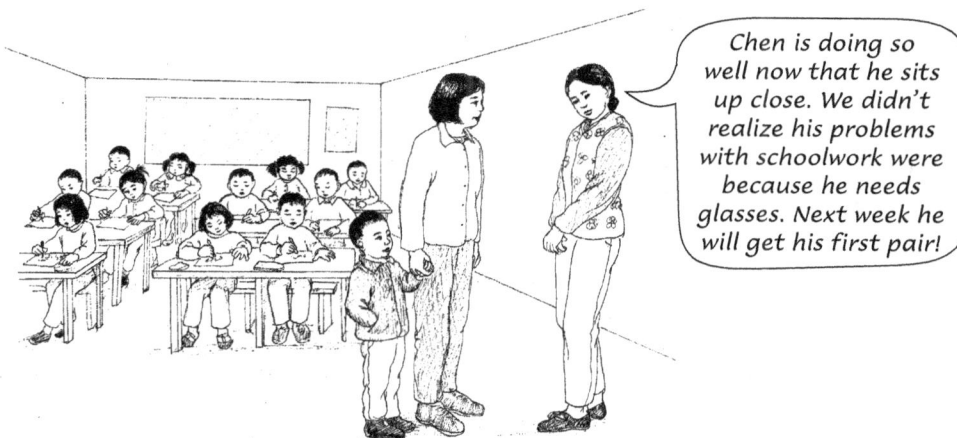

Chen is doing so well now that he sits up close. We didn't realize his problems with schoolwork were because he needs glasses. Next week he will get his first pair!

Eye Emergencies and Injuries

Some eye problems like injuries are clearly emergencies. Other eye problems may seem less urgent, such as signs of illness or infection, but if there are danger signs, they too can quickly lead to blindness.

Protect the eye (see page 12) and send the person to get emergency medical help for these danger signs:

DANGER SIGNS

- Sudden loss of vision in one or both eyes
- Any injury that cuts into the eyeball (page 9) or eyelid
- An injury with blood inside the colored part of the eye (page 10)
- Severe pain in the eye with a white-grayish spot on the clear part (cornea). Treat with antibiotic ointment (see pages 32 to 33) on the way to help. This could be an ulcer on the cornea (page 16).
- Severe pain inside the eye. This could be iritis (page 17) or acute glaucoma (page 20).
- Pus inside the colored part of the eye (page 10)
- In a baby or child, a cloudy or white pupil
- Seeing small spots (floaters, see page 23) are not an eye emergency unless they start suddenly along with flashes of light. This can happen when the retina, a part inside the eye, comes loose from the back of the eye. Surgery is needed soon to prevent loss of vision.
- Sudden double vision, especially in both eyes at once, can be a sign of several problems.

Also treat as an emergency any infection or inflammation that does not get better after 4 days of antibiotic ointment or drops.

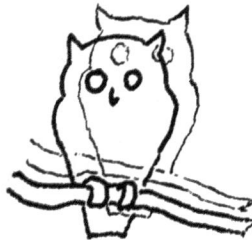

Double vision is seeing everything as if there were two. Suddenly seeing double may indicate a serious problem. Get medical help.

Injuries to the eye

Anything sharp or that can scratch the eye, such as thorns, branches, or pieces of metal from factory or other work, can seriously injure the eye. Treatment by an experienced health worker is important so injury does not lead to blindness. Even small scratches or cuts can get infected and harm vision if not cared for correctly. A wound inside the eyeball is especially dangerous.

If the eye has been hit hard with a fist, stone or other hard object, the eye is in danger. And if the eye becomes very painful 1 or 2 days after being hit, this could be acute glaucoma (page 20).

DANGER SIGNS

- The person cannot see well with the injured eye.
- There is a thorn, splinter, or other object stuck in the eye.
- The wound is deep.
- There is blood or pus inside the colored part of the eye.
- The pupils do not get smaller in response to brighter light.

TREATMENT

Apply an antibiotic eye drop if available and cover the eye by taping a paper cup over the eye, gently bandaging around the object, or using a cone made out of stiff paper (see page 12). Send the person for medical help.

If the person has none of these danger signs and can see well with the injured eye, apply antibiotic eye treatment (see pages 31 to 33), lightly cover the eye with a clean eye pad, and wait for a day or two. But if the eye does not improve, get medical help.

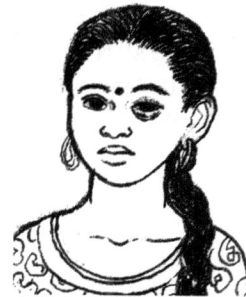

If you help a person who has been hit, try to find out if she was abused and is still in danger. Help people suffering violence in the home or workplace. See Chapter 18 in *Where Women Have No Doctor.*

Bleeding behind the cornea (hyphaema)

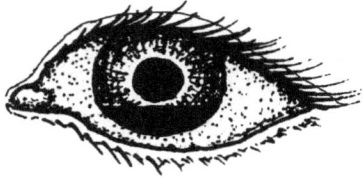

Blood pooling behind the cornea
is dangerous.

Blood in the colored part of the eye (the iris) is serious. The blood is trapped behind the clear covering (cornea) and may cover the iris. The person will not see well and may feel pain. The cause of this kind of bleeding is usually because the eye was hit with something hard, like a fist or stone. Send the person to an eye specialist right away. Have him sit upright on the way so that the bleeding does not block his vision.

If there is blood in the white part of the eye, usually it is not dangerous and will go away in a few weeks (see Blood in the white of the eye, page 21).

Pus behind the cornea (hypopyon)

Pus trapped between the clear covering (cornea) and the colored part of the eye (iris) is a sign that eye is in danger. The pus shows there is severe inflammation. This can occur because of an ulcer on the cornea or after eye surgery. Put antibiotic eye ointment in the eye (pages 31 to 33) and send the person for medical help right away.

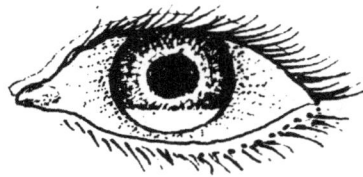

Injuries to the eye from chemicals

When cleaners, pesticides, gasoline (petrol) or other fuels, car battery acid, snake venom, lime powder (limestone), or other chemicals get into the eye, they can cause immediate injury so it is important to act quickly.

1. You will need lots of clean water to pour on the eye.

2. Have the person lie down.

3. The chemical may be trapped under the eyelid. Hold the eye or eyes open (the injured person or another person can help) as you gently pour the water onto the eye to rinse it.

4. As you wash the chemical out, don't let the water run from one eye into the other. If only one eye is affected, tilt the head so the water runs toward the side of the head, not toward the other eye. If the chemical went into both eyes, tilt the head back and pour the water on the nose so that it runs toward both eyes at the same time.

5. Keep pouring water gently over the eye or eyes for at least 15 minutes to 30 minutes. The chemical may still be causing harm to the eye even if it seems to have washed away.

6. After rinsing, put antibiotic ointment in the affected eye or eyes and send the person for medical help.

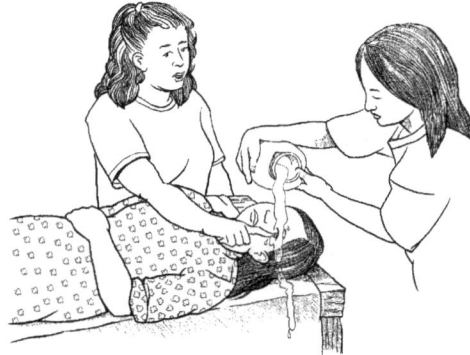

Police may use chemicals such as pepper spray and tear gas that irritate or harm eyes. Move away as best you can. The effect should wear off soon for tear gas and after an hour for pepper spray. Flush with water as described above.

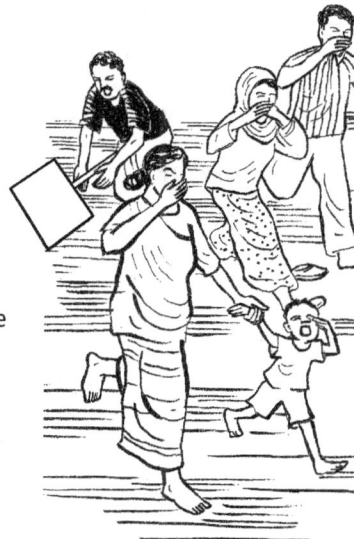

Protect eyes when injured or healing

After an injury, a paper cup or an eye cone can protect the eye while the person goes for emergency help. The eye cone will help remind the person not to rub her eye by mistake and can prevent the injury from getting worse.

Make an eye cone

1. Cut a circle out of a clean piece of heavy paper or thin cardboard.

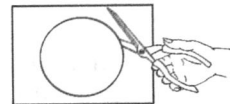

2. Cut into the middle in a straight line, and make a small hole in the middle.

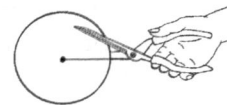

3. Make a cone shape.

4. Tape the cone, outside and inside.

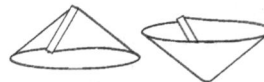

5. Tape the cone over the injured closed eye using tape that sticks well to skin.

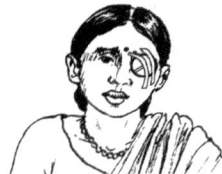

   If you cannot make an eye cone or the injury is not severe, use an eye pad. If a person had an operation, help change the eye pad often. If there are signs of infection, like redness and discharge, this is a sign the eye needs urgent treatment. In this case, covering the eye can make it worse.

Make an eye pad

1. Wash your hands well with soap and water.
2. Do not touch the eye with your hands.
3. Ask the person to shut both eyes while you cover the eye that needs the eye pad.
4. Cover the eye with sterile gauze or a very clean cloth cut into a square (6 centimeter sides).
5. Layer another 1 or 2 squares over the eye and use long strips of adhesive tape that sticks to skin to keep the eye pad in place.

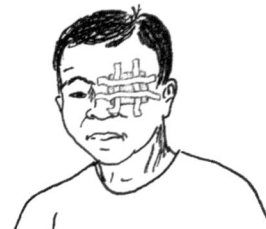

Red Eyes and Painful Eyes

Various problems cause red, painful eyes. When trying to determine the problem and what to do about it, ask the person if there was an injury to the eye or if he felt something go into the eyes.

Type of redness and pain	Possible cause
Usually **both eyes** but may start in **one eye** Mild burning pain Usually reddest at outer edges	If there is also thick white or yellow discharge, probably a bacterial infection called conjunctivitis (page 14) Trachoma (page 17) Measles
One or both eyes Redness and pain may be severe	An **injury** to the eye from something sharp or from a blow (page 9) Chemical burns or harmful liquids in the eye (page 11)
Usually **one eye only** Bleeding inside the eye, affecting the iris (colored part)	Bleeding in the colored part of the eye (page 10), often because of an **injury** This is an emergency.
Usually **one eye only** Redness and pain—not severe at first but can get worse	A bit of dirt in the eye (page 3) Scratch on the eye surface (page 16)
Usually **one eye only** Pain often severe Reddest close to the iris	Ulcer on the cornea (page 16) Iritis (page 17) Acute glaucoma (page 20) All are emergencies.
Usually **one eye only** Redness with a bump or swelling on the eyelid (with or without pain)	Infection around the eyelash or under the eyelid (page 22)
Usually **one eye only** Bright red patch on the white part of the eye	Probably a tiny blood vessel has burst, not an emergency (page 21)
Usually **both eyes** Discomfort but not pain Redness and itchy, watery eyes and sneezing, worse at certain seasons during the year	Hay fever, also called allergic conjunctivitis (page 16)
Usually **both eyes** Redness but no discharge and no pain Rash or fever	Conjunctivitis caused by a virus. If your region has Zika virus, red eyes could be one of the signs.

If there is redness, check if eyes are watery or have discharge (pus or secretions):

- Thick secretions or discharge can be conjunctivitis ('pink eye' or 'red eye'), a bacterial infection, especially if the eye is also very red.
- Watery eyes, with mild redness, that feel itchy in the corner of the eyes near the nose, are usually allergies.
- Watery eyes, with mild redness after a cold or flu, may be caused by a virus. This needs no special treatment and medicines will not help.
- Watery eyes, with redness and fever, cough and a runny nose, could be a sign of measles, even before a rash appears.

Conjunctivitis ('pink eye,' 'red eye')

Conjunctivitis can occur at any age, but is especially common in children.

SIGNS

- Eye looks pink or red
- Eye may itch or burn
- Starts in one eye, may spread to both
- Thick discharge may cause the eyelids to stick together overnight

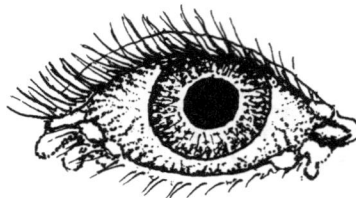

TREATMENT

Most conjunctivitis is caused by a virus that goes away in a few days without any special treatment.

If the yellow or white discharge is thick, the cause is likely a bacteria that can be treated with antibiotic eye ointment or drops (see Antibiotic eye treatments, pages 32 to 33). Even if the eye seems better, use the treatment for all 7 days so the infection does not come back.

Before applying antibiotic eye treatment, gently clean each eye with separate, wet cloths. Change cloths and wash your hands between cleaning and treating each eye to avoid spreading the infection from one eye to the other, or to yourself or other people.

PREVENTION

Conjunctivitis spreads very easily from one person to another. Wash hands often and after touching the eyes of another person or your own. Do not let a child with conjunctivitis use towels or bedding that others will use. Separate the child from other children until her eyes are better.

Conjunctivitis in newborn babies

An infection in a baby's eyes needs prompt treatment.

SIGNS

• Red, swollen eyes
• Pus in eyes
• Eyelids stuck together, especially upon waking

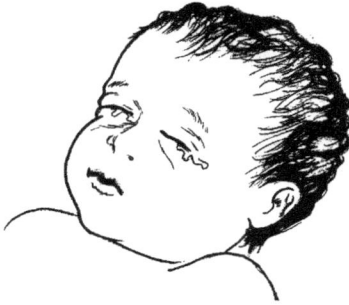

A newborn baby with red, swollen eyelids and pus may have an infection of gonorrhea or chlamydia that passed during birth. If eyes are swollen when the baby is between 2 and 4 days old, it is more likely to be gonorrhea. Treat immediately to prevent harm to the baby's eyes. If they are swollen when the baby is between 5 and 12 days old, it is more likely to be chlamydia. These infections, which spread during sex, affect many men and women but often give no signs of sickness. It is best to test and treat all pregnant women for these infections to prevent the baby from getting them at birth.

To protect the eyes from permanent damage and blindness, use antibiotic eye ointment (pages 32 to 33). Test the baby and mother to know what kind of infection they have. Both will need further treatment with antibiotics, not just eye ointment.

Care for a newborn baby's eyes to prevent problems

Immediately after birth, gently clean the baby's eyes with a new cotton swab. Then put antibiotic eye ointment on the eyes of a newborn baby to prevent eye infections. Use 1% tetracycline OR 0.5% to 1% erythromycin ointment. Put a thin line of ointment in each eye, 1 time only. Do this right away, within 2 hours after birth (see Antibiotic eye treatments, pages 32 to 33).

If a baby has watery eyes all the time, especially if tears fill the eye and run down the face even when the baby is not crying, it could be that the tiny tubes that drain tears away from the eye are blocked. This problem often goes away by itself, but a health worker can show you how to gently massage the baby's face on the side of the nose (Crigler or lacrimal sac massage), to help open the tubes.

Hay fever (allergic conjunctivitis) and allergies bothering the eyes

Dust, pollen, or other particles in the air cause sneezing along with red, itchy, and watery eyes in some people. When the body reacts with the same signs to the same thing every time, it is called an allergy. If this happens only certain times of the year, the person may have an allergy to pollen released by trees and plants (also called hay fever). If it happens all the time, the cause could be dust, mold, chemical products, or animals. Allergies irritate both eyes.

TREATMENT

If you know what is causing the eyes to react, the best treatment is to avoid or remove the source of the problem. For example:

- Try to keep sleeping areas and bedding free from dust. If an animal is causing the allergy, avoid the animal and the area where it sleeps.
- Close or cover windows at night.
- Use a dust mask or cloth to over your mouth and nose to protect yourself from breathing pollen and dust when working or walking outside.

Anything that is very close to your eye, like eye makeup, or something you can smell, such as clothing washed with perfumed soap, can also cause allergies that affect the eyes. If you stop using the product that is irritating your eyes, the allergy should bother you less.

Soothe itching eyes with a wet folded cloth over your eyes (cool water feels best). If antihistamine eye drops (see page 32) are available, they may help eyes feel better when hay fever is severe.

Ulcer on the cornea (damage to eye surface)

SIGNS

When the very delicate surface of the eye is damaged by infection or scratched, a painful corneal ulcer can result. Do not rub your eye, it only makes it worse.

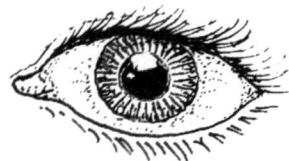

The person's vision is often reduced and they have severe pain. They may have thick or watery discharge.

The eye is red and if you look at the cornea in strong or bright light, you may see a gray-white patch. It may look less shiny than the rest of the eye.

TREATMENT

This is an emergency. If the ulcer on the cornea is not well cared for, it can cause blindness. Get medical help. Apply antibiotic eye ointment or drops in the affected eye every hour on the way to see an eye specialist (see pages 32 to 33).

Iritis (inflammation of the iris)

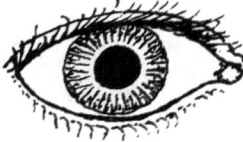

NORMAL EYE   EYE WITH IRITIS

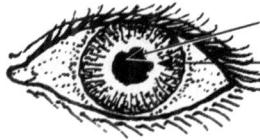

pupil small, often irregular

redness around iris

pain

Inflammation of the iris is called iritis. Its cause is usually not known.

SIGNS

• Usually in one eye only
• Deep aching pain in the eye
• The pupil (the black center of the eye) may have an irregular shape instead of round
• Redness on the white part of the eye closest to the iris
• The eye hurts more in bright light
• Vision is usually blurred

TREATMENT

Iritis is a serious eye problem and is painful. Get medical help within 1 to 2 days.

Antibiotics are not useful.

An experienced health worker may use eye drops to increase the size of the pupil, and other eye drops to decrease inflammation.

Trachoma — a chronic conjunctivitis

Trachoma is an eye infection that spreads from one person to another by hands, flies, and cloths that touched an infected eye. Trachoma is most common in children and their mothers. If a person is infected many times, after several years this can make the eyelashes turn in and scratch the eye's surface, which causes pain and loss of vision. Because it feels scratchy, it is sometimes called "hair in the eye."

Trachoma has become less common in the world but is still a serious problem in some countries, especially in Sub-Saharan Africa. It mostly affects people who live in poverty, in crowded conditions, and where there are many flies and little water. Improving water and sanitation is important in preventing trachoma.

SIGNS

- Trachoma often begins in young children like a mild conjunctivitis that is not very noticeable at first.
- Repeated infections in young children cause small white-gray swellings to form inside the upper eyelids. To see these, fold the eyelid back (see page 3).
- After years of repeated infections, these swellings or bumps become white scars under the eyelid. Scars pull the eyelashes inward and these scratch the clear part of the eye, causing pain to the eye and loss of vision.

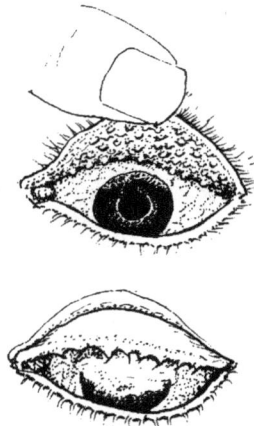

TREATMENT

The best treatment for trachoma is a single dose of azithromycin (page 34) by mouth. If azithromycin is not available, 1% tetracycline eye ointment inside the eye 2 times a day for 6 weeks also works.

For people with advanced trachoma, a simple surgery can make the turned-in eyelashes turn outward again. If surgery is not available, a trained eye-health worker may be able to remove the irritating eyelashes.

PREVENTION

Early and complete treatment of trachoma prevents its spread to other people. Wash children's faces every day and wash your hands after touching anyone's eyes. Wash towels, clothes, and bedding often to be sure that 2 people never share a pillow or the same cloth to dry their faces.

Keep flies away by covering food, keeping latrines covered, and composting away from the house. See Water and Sanitation: Keys to Staying Healthy.

If there are many cases in your community, health authorities may treat everyone in the community with azithromycin to stop trachoma from spreading.

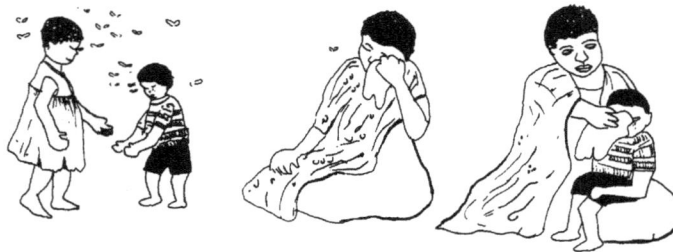

Trachoma is spread by flies, fingers, and fabric.

Common Eye Problems

Cataracts

The lens is a clear part inside the eye that focuses the light from outside so the eye can see. As people get older, the lens can become cloudy, blocking light from shining through it, and leading to a gradual loss of vision and eventual blindness. This cloudiness can sometimes be seen as a gray spot on the eye, called a cataract. Cataracts are most common in older people, but may occur in babies and children.

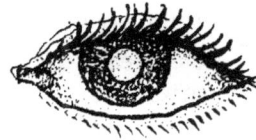

To delay the development of cataracts:

• Don't smoke.

• Wear hats to protect the eyes from strong sunlight.

Health workers can identify people with cataracts and recommend programs and hospitals that offer operations to restore sight. Women are less likely than men to get treatment for cataracts. Visit older women in their homes and ask about their eyesight. Checking older people can help them get treated before cataracts block their vision. But even if they can barely see, it is never too late to get them help.

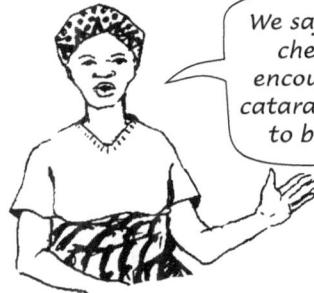

We say: "If there is gray hair, check for gray eyes." We encourage older people with cataracts to get the operation to bring back their vision.

TREATMENT

Medicines do not help a cataract go away. An operation removes the cataract (the cloudy lens) and puts in a clear lens so the person can see again.

After the operation, the person will need antibiotic and anti-inflammatory eye drops to help the eye heal, usually for about 4 weeks. The eye may be slightly uncomfortable and seeing can be blurred at first, but this should improve a little each day. If pain in the eye develops in the first two weeks, this is a danger sign. Get help from an eye doctor within 24 hours. Reading glasses may be needed after the operation in order to see close up.

When eye health programs come to the community

Doctors from your country or elsewhere may organize events to remedy eye problems, including operations to treat cataracts. Community leaders can work with the doctors to benefit as many people as possible. The helping group should provide:

- clear explanations to local health workers on how to care for the eyes after the operation.
- the eye drops that people will need to heal.
- information on where people can get eyeglasses, if needed, after the eyes have healed.
- who to contact if a problem arises after the operation, both in their organization and locally.

Glaucoma

Sometimes pressure increases inside the eye and damages nerves inside the eye, causing a serious disease called glaucoma. A person with glaucoma loses side vision and gradually can become blind. The eye may hurt and get hard like a marble. Glaucoma may be caused by an injury, but most often the cause is unknown.

A person with glaucoma needs treatment to lower the pressure. This may be eye drops daily for the rest of their life, or sometimes laser treatment or an operation is used to lower the eye pressure.

Glaucoma mostly affects people who are older than 40, especially those who have had a family member with glaucoma. Help people over 40 get their eyes checked for glaucoma every few years.

There are different forms of glaucoma. Most common are acute glaucoma and chronic glaucoma.

Acute glaucoma (angle-closure glaucoma)

This worsens very quickly. It causes a red and very painful eye with loss of vision. The person may feel nausea, have a headache, and their eye hurts more in bright light. The eye may feel hard compared to the other, normal eye. If not treated, acute glaucoma will cause blindness within a few days. Send the person for medical help immediately. They will first need eye drops that lower the pressure in the eye. Then they will likely need laser treatment or an operation.

Chronic glaucoma (open-angle glaucoma)

In chronic glaucoma, the pressure in both eyes increases slowly over months and years. There is no pain. Side (peripheral) vision is lost first. As the glaucoma gets worse, it is like looking through a tunnel. The person often does not notice until vision loss is severe. Eye doctors can test side vision and look inside the eye to check for this kind of glaucoma. The earlier it is treated, the better. Treatment with eye drops, laser, or surgery can stop vision from getting worse.

Fleshy growth across eye (pterygium)

A fleshy thickening on the eye surface that slowly grows out from the white part of the eye near the nose and toward the middle is called a pterygium. It is common and usually not serious. People who spend many years working outside in strong sunlight or where there is wind or dust are more likely to have them.

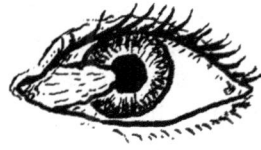

Wearing dark glasses and hats helps keep sunlight, wind, and dust away from the eyes, which prevents or slows the growth.

Often these need no treatment. If it is too close to the colored part of the eye or causes too much discomfort, the growth can be removed by an eye surgeon before it begins to affect the person's vision.

Blood in the white of the eye

Blood in the white of the eye occasionally appears after lifting something heavy, coughing hard, or a minor injury to the eye. It results from the bursting of a tiny blood vessel. It is harmless, like a bruise, and it will slowly disappear on its own within 2 weeks. No treatment is needed.

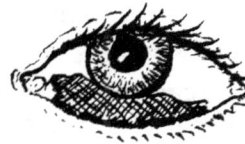

A patch of blood in the white part is usually harmless.

However, if blood is in the colored part of the eye (the iris), this is serious. See page 10.

Dry eyes and crusty eyelids

Dry eyes are caused by dry climates, getting older, smoke in the air, and some medications.

Crusty eyelids can happen when dirt or discharge blocks moisture and tears, making eyes dry and itchy. The person may get eyelid infections (see below) or crust or dandruff-like flakes along the eyelid. When the eyelids and face around the eyes are clean, the tears and natural moisture of the eyes can keep them healthy.

TREATMENT

For dry eyes, rest your eyes by closing them now and then. If your eyes stay dry, you can try warm compresses 1 to 2 times a day for 5 to 10 minutes to increase the natural moisture in the eyes. Lubricating eye drops can also help (see page 32).

For crust on the eyelids, use warm compresses 2 to 4 times a day, followed by a gentle washing of the eyelids. If it does not improve, there may be a bacterial infection and you can try erythromycin antibiotic eye ointment 2 times a day for 7 days (see Antibiotic eye treatments, page 32).

Lumps and swelling on the eyelids

A red swollen lump on the eyelid usually is either:

- a stye, a painful lump caused by an infection around an eyelash; or
- a chalazion, a lump that may not hurt, caused by blockage inside the eyelid.

Sometimes an infection that starts around an eyelash can spread to inside the eyelid.

Both can be treated with warm compresses 4 times a day for 15 or 20 minutes each time. Re-heat the cloth several times while using to keep it as warm as possible without burning. Do not squeeze or puncture the lump as this makes the problem worse.

If swelling does not lessen in a few days, get medical help.

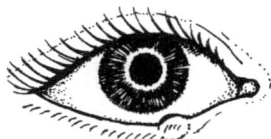

A stye is a painful infection around the eyelash.

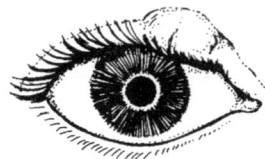

A lump under the eyelid that does not hurt may be a chalazion.

Floaters (seeing small spots)

Floaters or small moving spots are sometimes seen when looking at a bright surface (like a wall or the sky). The spots move when the eyes move and look like tiny flies. These spots are common and usually harmless.

If large numbers of floating spots appear suddenly and vision begins to fail in one eye, or you also continue to see flashes of light, this could be a sign of a condition called a detached retina. A surgery at an eye hospital is needed as soon as possible to reattach the retina.

Vitamin A deficiency (night blindness, xerophthalmia)

Lack of vitamin A is a type of malnutrition that can damage the eyes of children, causing blindness. This is preventable.

Protect the eyes of small children by making sure they eat foods rich with vitamin A, including orange foods such as carrots, mango, and papaya, and green leafy vegetables, fish, and eggs. Breastfeeding helps protect a baby's eyes from lack of vitamin A along with providing many other benefits for the baby's health.

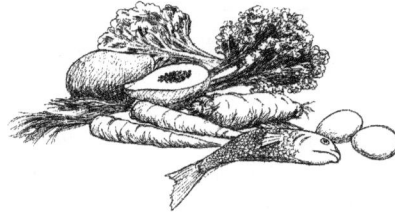

Where this type of malnutrition is common, sometimes all children are given a vitamin A supplement every 6 months (page 34).

SIGNS

First, the eyes become dry and produce less tears. Then there is more difficulty seeing in dim light. The white part of the eye loses its shine and starts to wrinkle. Eventually the eyes become more damaged and the child may become blind.

TREATMENT

If a child cannot see well in the evening or if the child has measles, then treat the child with vitamin A (page 34).

Crossed eyes, wandering eye, squint (strabismus)

If one or both eyes of a baby or a child do not look straight, this condition can lead to a loss of vision in the wandering eye. Get the child to an eye specialist. It is not an emergency, but the child should go as young as possible to have the best chance of correcting his vision.

TREATMENT

The eye doctor may patch the good eye to make the wandering eye work better or prescribe special glasses to help. An operation can usually straighten the eye but is often not necessary.

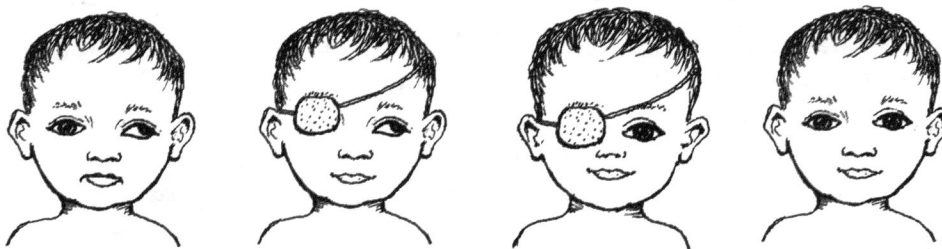

Sometimes patching the good eye will help the wandering eye become straight and better at seeing. Some children need the patch a few hours a day and some will need to wear it all day.

Pregnancy and vision

Changes in hormones can cause a woman's vision to change during pregnancy, but usually after the baby is born her vision goes back to the way it was.

Pregnant women who suddenly have blurred vision, see spots, lose vision in one eye, or have double vision could be having danger signs of a serious condition called pre-eclampsia. Pre-eclampsia also brings headaches and high blood pressure (140/90 or higher). Get help right away.

Help pregnant women get tested for gonorrhea and chlamydia and to receive treatment if they need it. Women can have either of these illnesses that are passed during sex and not know it. If these germs spread to the baby's eyes during birth, the baby can lose her sight.

Protect pregnant women from rubella and Zika, illnesses that can cause serious eye problems in babies. Rubella (German measles) is prevented by a vaccine.

Illnesses that Can Affect the Eyes

Some infections or illnesses affecting the whole body can harm the eyes. When someone has eye problems, it is wise to consider if the cause could be another illness.

Tuberculosis can infect the eyes and cause redness or poor vision. Most often, signs of tuberculosis will appear first in the lungs or other parts of the body.

HIV and AIDS: Eye problems and loss of vision in people with HIV are prevented by treatment with HIV medicines, called ART. Get tested so you can start treatment if you need it.

Herpes (cold sores) occasionally spreads to the eye, causing an ulcer of the cornea with pain, blurred vision, and watery eyes. Antiviral medicines are helpful. Do not use steroid eye drops—they make the problem worse.

Problems in the liver: Jaundice, when the white part of the eye is yellow (or the skin of a light-colored person gets yellow), can be a sign of hepatitis.

Diabetes and high blood pressure

People with diabetes may develop vision problems. As the disease advances, diabetes can damage their eyes (a serious condition called diabetic retinopathy). Without treatment, diabetes can lead to blindness. Blurred vision can be an early sign that blood sugar is high and a person may have diabetes. If someone with blurred vision also is very thirsty and has to urinate a lot, it is likely they have diabetes. Inexpensive tests can let them know for sure.

Help people with diabetes get treatment to bring down their blood sugar levels and encourage them to visit an eye specialist once a year to check their eyes for damage from diabetes. Eye disease from diabetes can be treated if found early.

High blood pressure can affect the eyes and vision by damaging the blood vessels inside the eye. Checking blood pressure during health care visits is the best way to know if it is too high. Preventing and treating high blood pressure will help protect the eyes.

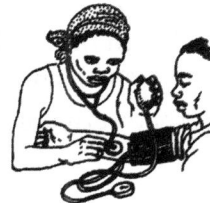

River blindness (onchocerciasis)

This disease of the eyes and skin is becoming less common. It is still found in parts of Africa, Yemen, and a few communities in the Amazon region of South America. River blindness is caused by tiny worms that are carried by black flies. The worms get inside a person when an infected fly bites him.

The black fly has a humped back like this

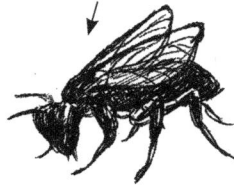

but is actually much smaller, like this.

SIGNS

- Itchy skin and rash
- 2 to 3 cm lumps you can feel under the skin

Without treatment, the skin gradually becomes wrinkled and loose. White spots and patches may appear on the front of the lower legs.

The illness can lead to eye problems and sometimes blindness. First there may be redness and watery eyes, then signs of iritis may follow (page 17).

TREATMENT

The medicine ivermectin treats river blindness. Where ivermectin is given every 6 months or once a year as part of community-wide campaigns, fewer people get the disease and it may disappear from the region.

PREVENTION

- These black flies breed in fast-running water. Clearing brush from the edges of stream and river banks helps reduce their number.
- Avoid sleeping outside, especially in the daytime when the flies bite most.
- Cooperate with programs working to lower the number of black flies and with the health workers giving ivermectin to the whole community to prevent new cases.

Early treatment prevents blindness and reduces spread of the disease.

Poor Vision and Eyeglasses

Many children and adults do not see well. A person may not see people or read signs clearly from far away or must squint to see up close. They may have headaches or blurred vision after reading before realizing they need eyeglasses. With eyeglasses matched to your eyes, you can see better. See if there are programs where you live that test vision and supply free or low-cost eyeglasses.

Before I didn't want Sarita to use the glasses too often because I worried they would break, but now I know she must wear them all day so she can see.

It is common for a person's vision to change. You may need to change your eyeglasses every few years.

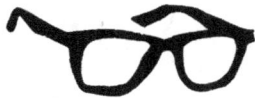

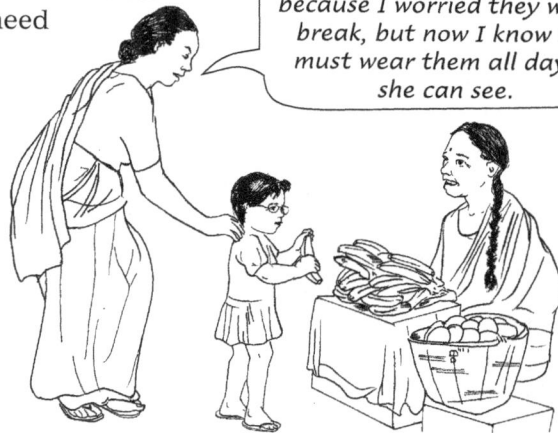

Testing sight for distance vision

Check vision with an 'E' chart (found at the end of this booklet). Test each eye separately by having the person cover the other eye with the palm of their hand or thick paper. The person looks at each row and uses their free hand or a paper 'E' to show if the bars on the 'E' point up, down, or to one side. The row with the smallest size of letters they see well is the measure of their eyesight. For example, if the person can read most of the row of letters labeled 6/12 but less than half of the row of smaller letters after that, we say they have 6/12 vision.

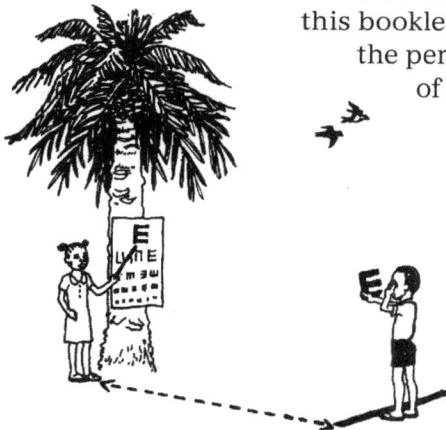

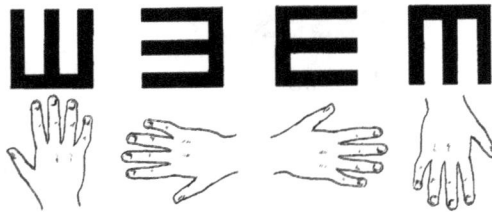

Use your hand to point the same way
as the bars on the 'E.'

For an adult, if distance vision is poor (they cannot read the 6/18 or smaller letters on the eye chart), send them to an eye doctor. For school children, check to make sure they can read the 6/12 line letters. Sometimes a child does not do well in school only because she cannot see clearly from far away. Eyeglasses will help her learn.

'E' charts are made in different sizes to be used at 6 meters, 3 meters, or other distances. There are also mobile phone applications that make an 'E' of different sizes to do the same test without a chart. For the test to be accurate, follow the instructions carefully for the chart or phone app you are using. Carefully measure the correct distance where the person needs to stand.

Use the 'E' chart, found at the end of this booklet, with the person standing 3 meters away from the chart.

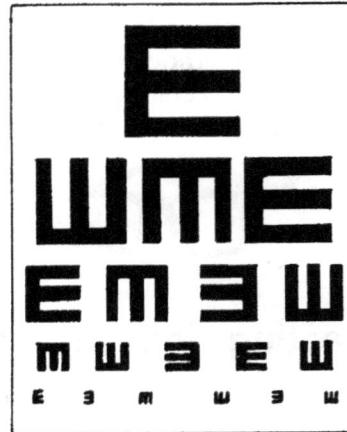

There are 2 ways of writing how well the person sees based on an eye chart test. The number sets showing 20/200, 20/20 etc. begin with the number 20 because 20 feet is the distance for a larger eye chart. Using meters, the numbers are 6/60, 6/6 etc. because 6 meters is about 20 feet. Any chart or measure system you use will likely have one of these 2 number systems to label the different rows even if the chart is meant to be used at distance other than 20 feet or 6 meters. The better the eyesight, the lower the second number:

> 6/18 = 20/60: An adult sees well enough for most work
>
> 6/12 = 20/40: A child sees well enough for school
>
> 6/6 = 20/20: The person sees very well

Reading glasses

People over the age of 40 years may have a harder time seeing well enough to do close-up tasks like reading, sorting seeds, or threading a needle. Reading glasses magnify close-up things to look larger. They come in several different strengths of magnification. Glasses that are labeled +1 make close objects look slightly bigger, +2 make them look even bigger, and +3 the biggest. Test each of the different reading glasses by trying to read a book or thread a needle at a comfortable distance.

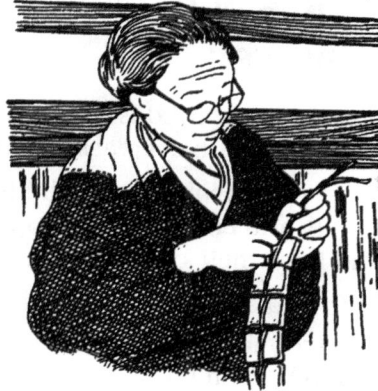

If a person has trouble seeing close up and also cannot see well far away, reading glasses may not solve the problem. Help them visit an eye clinic to find out what is affecting their vision.

Contact lenses and surgery to correct vision

Contact lenses are tiny plastic lenses that rest directly on the eye to correct vision, just as eyeglasses do. After a vision test, a specialist can help you find contact lenses that will work for your eyes. Do not use contact lenses made for someone else. Do not sleep wearing contact lenses unless they are made for overnight use. There are many different kinds of contact lenses and each needs specific liquids to disinfect, store and rinse them. Do not use homemade versions of the contact lens liquids.

While contact lenses are convenient, they can cause serious problems if not cared for and used properly. To prevent infections, always wash your hands before touching contact lenses. If you have mild irritation in your eye or an eye infection, do not use contact lenses until your eyes are better. Clean and disinfect lenses before wearing them again. If a contact lens has a torn edge, do not use it. If you have pain, burning, discharge, unusual redness, or blurred vision, this could be a danger sign of a scratch or ulcer on the cornea (page 16) or another serious problem. Get help from an experienced health worker.

For some people, poor vision can be repaired with laser surgery (surgery using a very strong beam of light instead of cutting instruments). This is different than the kind of surgery to treat cataracts and may be expensive. Before spending money, it is wise to talk to others who have used the same eye surgeon with good results.

People with blindness or poor vision that cannot be improved

Sometimes a child is born blind or a person's poor vision cannot be improved with eyeglasses, surgery, or medicines.

People learn to live with blindness and poor vision. With support from family and community, people who are blind attend school, earn a living, and have their own families.

To make life easier and safer for a person with poor vision or blindness:

- Introduce yourself when speaking to the person, speak to him directly and let him know when you are walking away from him.

- Let him grasp your elbow when you walk together. You can alert him and lead him around any danger. This is a more respectful than pulling a person along by his hand or body.

- Create handrails or guide ropes to the latrine or other places the person goes to daily.

- Do not move furniture or other objects to a different place in the home, school or workplace. Alert the person if you do move something.

- Drive carefully in the area where a blind person lives. A bell on a cow or other animal warns a person who does not see.

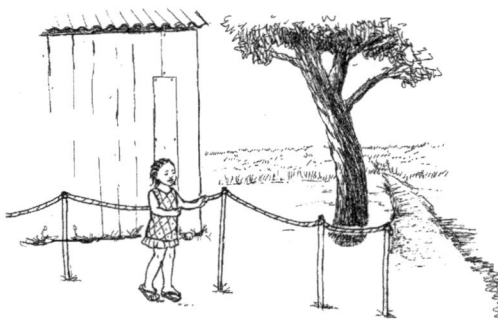

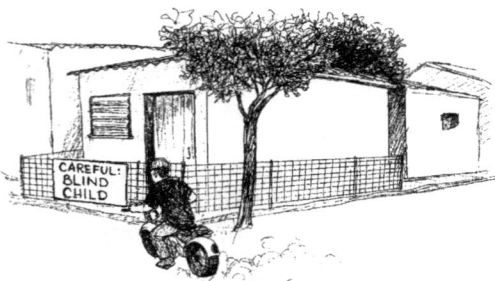

Children with disabilities, including blindness, can be more at risk for abuse, including sexual abuse, than children who can see. They need family and community protection to keep them safe, especially while young.

See the Hesperian book *Helping Children Who Are Blind* to learn more about how young children with vision problems can learn to take care of themselves, go to school, and lead good lives. Helping children to move about, understand the world around them and learn the skills they need is very important. See *A Health Handbook for Women with Disabilities* for ideas about how health workers, families, and communities can support everyone with disabilities to have better lives and better health.

Problems with the Eyes and Seeing: Medicines

How to use eye ointment or eye drops

Wash your hands before and after applying eye drops or eye ointment because many eye infections spread easily through touching a person's face and then your own eye. Eye drop bottles come with a seal. Help the person break the seal and show them how to squeeze out 1 drop.

To be effective, eye drops and ointment must go inside—not outside—the eyelid. Ointment will last longer in the eye and work well overnight but will blur vision temporarily making drops more convenient during the day.

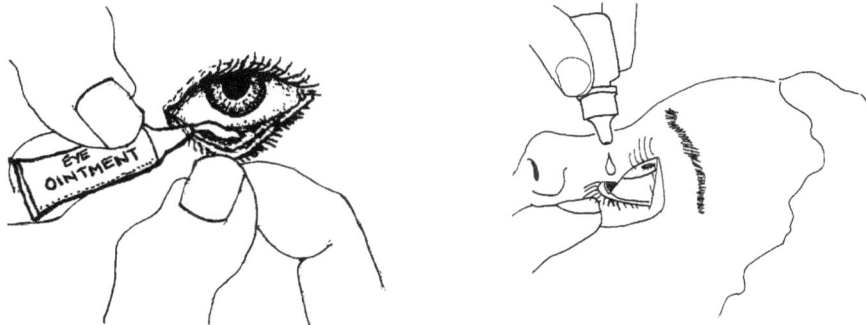

To avoid spreading germs, do not let the tube or the dropper touch the eye.

To use eye ointment, gently pull down the lower eyelid and squeeze a thin line of ointment along the length of the eye, starting at the inner corner.

To use eye drops, pull out the lower eyelid to make a small pouch and gently squeeze 1 to 2 drops into it while looking up. Gently close your eye but try not to blink. Most of the drop will spread around the eye surface.

Common types of eye drops

Eye drops with antibiotics are used to treat an infection by germs (bacteria). Eye antibiotics also come as ointments. Antibiotic eye drops and ointments will not help irritated or red eyes caused by a virus.

Eye drops with antihistamines relieve watery, red, and itching eyes caused by allergies. Cold compresses on the eyes can help calm itching eyes and cost nothing.

Eye drops for lubrication, called "artificial tears" or "natural tears," are used for eyes that feel dry. They can be used up to 4 times a day and at night just before sleep. Resting with warm compresses over closed eyes 1 to 2 times a day for 5 to 10 minutes can help your eyes make more of their own moisture.

Eye drops with natamycin are sometimes used by health workers to prevent fungal infections when there is an ulcer on the cornea.

Eye drops with tetrahydrozoline or naphzoline shrink the tiny blood vessels so the eyes look less red. Because they do not cure the cause of a red eye, they are a waste of money.

Important ⚠

Eye drops with steroids (such as prednisolone or dexamethasone) reduce eye inflammation after surgery or from some other eye diseases. If used incorrectly, steroid eye drops can cause severe harm to the eye or may hide a problem that needs other treatment. Some drops mix antibiotics and steroids (often adding 'Dex' or 'Pred' to the name). Use eye drops with steroids only when specifically recommended by an experienced health worker.

Antibiotic eye treatments

Antibiotic eye treatments have the word "eye" or "ophthalmic" on the label to show they are safe for use in the eye. Do not use antibiotic skin ointments in the eyes.

Antibiotic eye ointment and antibiotic eye drops treat eye infections caused by bacteria and treat ulcers on the cornea. Erythromycin or tetracycline eye ointment is used at birth to protect a newborn baby's eyes from infections that may pass at birth.

Common antibiotic eye treatments include:

- 1% tetracycline eye ointment
- 0.5% or 1% erythromycin eye ointment
- 0.3% ciprofloxacin eye drops or ointment
- 0.3% ofloxacin eye drops
- 0.3% gentamycin eye drops
- 10% sulfacetamide eye drops
- 0.5% chloramphenicol eye drops

How to use

For an eye drop or an eye ointment to work, it must be put inside—not outside—the eyelid. Show the person you are helping how to use them (see page 31).

FOR CONJUNCTIVITIS (PINK EYE) CAUSED BY BACTERIA

Use the antibiotic eye ointment or antibiotic eye drops 4 times a day for 7 days in both eyes. Even if the eye seems better, use the antibiotic treatment for all 7 days so that the infection does not come back. Sometimes it takes 2 days for the medicine to start working.

FOR AN ULCER ON THE CORNEA

Apply antibiotic eye drops every hour and send the person for help. The drops are applied every hour for 24 hours and then, if improving, drops are applied 4 times a day for 7 days. More advanced help is needed if the eye does not improve in 2 days. For an ulcer on the cornea, never use drops or ointment that contain steroids.

FOR TRACHOMA

If azithromycin pills (page 34) are not available, tetracycline antibiotic eye ointment can be used. Use 1% tetracycline antibiotic eye ointment in both eyes, 2 times a day every day for 6 weeks.

FOR NEWBORN BABIES TO PREVENT EYE PROBLEMS

Antibiotics are used to protect the newborn baby's eyes from infection that can pass to the baby during birth.

After gently wiping the eyelids with a cloth and water immediately after birth, use one of these antibiotic ointments with every newborn baby in both eyes within the first 2 hours:

1% tetracycline OR **0.5% to 1% erythromycin ointment** Put a thin line of ointment in each eye, 1 time only, within 2 hours after the birth.

➡ Gently pull down the lower eyelid and squeeze a thin line of ointment along the eye moving from the inside corner outward (see page 31). Do not let the tube touch the baby's eye and do not wipe the ointment away.

If there is no ointment, use:

2.5% solution of povidone-iodine

➡ Put 1 drop in each eye, 1 time only, within 2 hours of birth.

Pull down the lower eyelid and squeeze 1 drop into this pocket (see page 31). Do not let the dropper touch the eye.

Azithromycin

Azithromycin is an antibiotic that treats many infections including trachoma, for which just 1 dose by mouth is needed. Where health authorities have campaigns to eliminate trachoma, azithromycin may be offered to the whole community to cure current infections of trachoma and prevent new ones at the same time.

How to use

FOR TRACHOMA

➡ **Children 6 months and older, up to 40 kg.** To dose by weight: give at least 20 mg per kg by mouth in a single dose, but do not give more than 1000 mg (1 g).

For young children, liquid azithromycin is mixed to a strength of 200 mg/5 ml. For example, a child weighing 10 kg would take a single 5 ml dose (200 mg).

Give older children azithromycin by mouth. Pills usually come in 250 mg. It is safe to give a little more instead of dividing pills in half. For example, give 500 mg for children that weigh between 20 kg and 30 kg. Give 750 mg for children that weigh between 30 kg and 40 kg.

Programs distributing azithromycin often determine the dose based on the height of the child.

➡ **Young people that weigh over 40 kg and adults (including pregnant women):** give 1000 mg (1 g) by mouth in a single dose. Taking 4 pills that each have 250 mg is the same as 1 g.

When azithromycin is given to the whole community for prevention, doses may be given once every year for 3 years.

If azithromycin by mouth is not available, trachoma can be treated with antibiotic eye ointment. Use 1% tetracycline antibiotic eye ointment in both eyes, 2 times a day every day for 6 weeks.

Vitamin A, retinol

Vitamin A prevents night blindness and xerophthalmia.

To get enough vitamin A, people need to eat enough yellow fruits and vegetables, dark green leafy vegetables, and foods such as eggs, fish, and liver. In areas where night blindness and xerophthalmia are common and eating enough of these foods is not always possible, give children vitamin A every 6 months.

Important ⚠

Do not use more than the suggested amount. Too much vitamin A from capsules, tablets, or oil can be dangerous. Do not give the regular adult dose of 200,000 U to girls or women who could become pregnant, or women in the first 3 months of pregnancy because this can harm a developing baby. For pregnant women, vitamin A is given in smaller doses more often instead of a single large dose.

How to use

Swallow pills or capsules. But for young children, crush tablets and mix them with a little breast milk. Or cut open capsules and squeeze the liquid into the child's mouth.

TO PREVENT VITAMIN A DEFICIENCY IN CHILDREN

As part of a prevention program:

➡ **6 months to 1 year:** give 100,000 U by mouth one time.
Over 1 year: give 200,000 U by mouth one time. Repeat every 6 months.

TO TREAT NIGHT BLINDNESS

If someone already has difficulty seeing or has other signs of night blindness, 3 doses are given. The first dose is given right away, the second is given one day later and the third dose at least 2 weeks later.

➡ For each of the 3 doses:
Under 6 months: give 50,000 U by mouth in each dose.
6 months to 1 year: give 100,000 U by mouth in each dose.
Over 1 year: give 200,000 U by mouth in each dose.

➡ **For pregnant women:** give 25,000 U by mouth weekly in pregnancy for 12 weeks. If she has continued signs of night blindness or another severe eye problem from lack of vitamin A, an experienced health worker may give a pregnant woman a larger dose.

FOR CHILDREN WITH MEASLES

Vitamin A can help prevent pneumonia and blindness – two common complications of measles.

➡ **Under 6 months:** give 50,000 U by mouth 1 time a day for 2 days.
6 months to 1 year: give 100,000 U by mouth 1 time a day for 2 days.
Over 1 year: give 200,000 U by mouth 1 time a day for 2 days.

If the child has already received a dose of vitamin A in the last 6 months, give this treatment for one day only. If someone with measles is severely malnourished or already starting to lose her vision, give a third dose of vitamin A after 2 weeks.

Where To Get More Information

Additional resources on eye health that Hesperian and Seva recommend:

- *Community Eye Health Journal* –search by topic or look through articles. These often include photos of eye conditions. https://cehjournal.org/
- These posters show how to identify and treat common eye conditions: https://www.cehjournal.org/resources/primary-level-management-eye-injury-trauma/ and https://www.cehjournal.org/resources/primary-level-management-red-eye-no-injury/
- Migrant Clinician's Network's *Primary Eye Care Manual for Migrant Farmworkers and Their Families*. https://www.migrantclinician.org/files/resourcebox/Eyecare.pdf
- World Health Organization, Africa, *Primary Eye Care Training Manual*. https://www.afro.who.int/sites/default/files/2018-06/WEB-2835-OMS-Afro-PrimaryEyeCaretrainingmanual-20180406.pdf
- The Fred Hollows Foundation's list of common eye condition terms and their meaning. https://www.hollows.org/au/eye-health-glossary
- Aravind Eye Care System offers free short courses on eye care: http://www.aurosiksha.org/

Thanks

We are grateful for input and feedback from everyone within Hesperian and many individuals and organizations worldwide:

Research, writing and editing: Christine Chmielewski, Paula Worby, Todd Jailer.

Design: Kathleen Tandy.

Group reviews convened by: Aravind Eye Care System, India; Centre for Community Medicine and Primary Healthcare, Nmandi Azikiwe University, Nigeria; Community Based Initiatives in Health, Water and Sanitation (COBIHESA), Tanzania; Comprehensive Rural Health Project (CRHP), Jamkhed, India; Hillside Health Care International, Belize; Kilimanjaro Centre for Community Ophthalmology (KCCO), Tanzania.

Additional review and consultation: Jordan Kasselow, David Katusabe, Joseph Michon, Siddharth Narendran, Matthew Nicasio, Raymond Okechukwu, Scott Pike, Noela Prasad, Dhivya Ramasamy, Fortunate Shija, Chundak Tenzing, Alasana Touray, Ashok Vardhan. Special thanks to Allen Foster of the International Centre for Eye Health, London School of Hygiene & Tropical Medicine.

Illustrations: Akiko Aoyagi Shurtleff, Heidi Broner, Regina Doyle, Victoria Francis, Jesse Hamm, Haris Ichwan, Anna Kallis, June Mehra, Naoko Miyamoto, Kate Peatman, Kathleen Tandy, David Werner, Mary Ann Zapalac, Victor Zubeldía.

Distance vision acuity eye chart design: Matthew Smith.

Other Titles from Hesperian Health Guides:

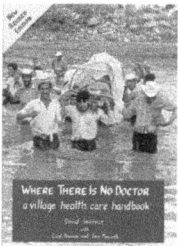

Where There Is No Doctor, by David Werner, Carol Thuman and Jane Maxwell, is the most widely used health manual in the world with information on how to diagnose, treat and prevent common diseases, emphasizing prevention and the importance of community mobilization. 512 pages.

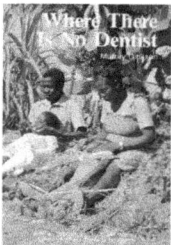

Where There Is No Dentist, by Murray Dickson, shows how to care for teeth and gums at home, and in community and school settings. Detailed, illustrated information on dental equipment, placing fillings and pulling teeth, teaching hygiene and nutrition, and HIV and oral health. 248 pages.

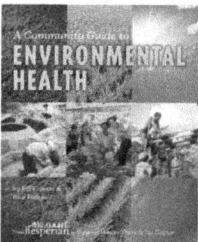

A Community Guide to Environmental Health, by Jeff Conant and Pam Fadem, helps urban and rural health promoters, activists and community leaders take charge of environmental health from toilets to toxics, watershed management to waste management, and agriculture to air pollution. Includes activities, how-to instructions, and stories. 640 pages.

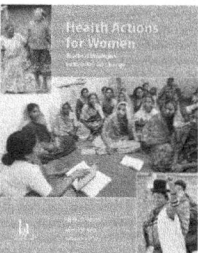

Health Actions for Women, by Melissa Smith, Sarah Shannon and Kathleen Vickery, was field tested by 41 community-based groups in 23 countries and provides a wealth of clearly explained and engagingly illustrated activities, strategies and stories that address the social obstacles and practices that prevent women and girls from enjoying healthy lives. 352 pages.

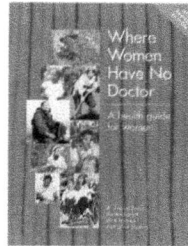

Where Women Have No Doctor, by A. August Burns, Ronnie Lovich, Jane Maxwell and Katharine Shapiro, combines self-help medical information with an understanding of the ways poverty, discrimination and cultural beliefs limit women's health and access to care. Clearly written and with over 1000 drawings, this is an essential resources for any woman who wants to improve her health. 600 pages.

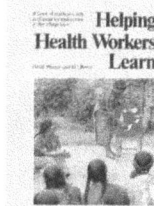

Helping Health Workers Learn, by David Werner and Bill Bower, is an indispensable resource that makes health education fun and effective. Includes activities, techniques, and ideas for low-cost teaching aids, and presents strategies for community involvement through participatory education. 640 pages.

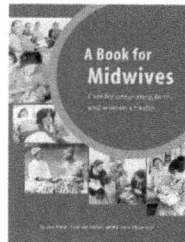

A Book for Midwives, by Susan Klein, Suellen Miller and Fiona Thomson, is an invaluable training tool and practical reference for midwives and anyone concerned about care for women in pregnancy, birth and beyond. This book discusses preventing, managing and treating obstetric complications, covers HIV in pregnancy, birth and breastfeeding, and has extensive information on reproductive care. 544 pages.

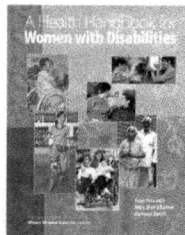

A Health Handbook for Women with Disabilities, by Jane Maxwell, Julia Watts Belser and Darlena David. This handbook provides groundbreaking advice and suggestions from women with disabilities worldwide, and helps women with disabilities improve their health, self-esteem, and ability to care for themselves and participate in their communities. 416 pages.

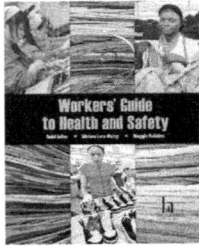

Workers' Guide to Health and Safety, by Todd Jailer, Miriam Lara-Meloy and Maggie Robbins, shows how workers can assess their workplaces, recognize hazards, and take charge of their health and safety, especially in electronics, shoe, and garment factories. Focuses on developing actionable alternatives to hazardous conditions and organizing for improvements. 576 pages.

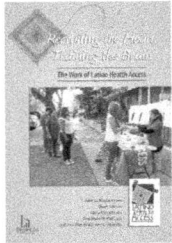

Recruiting the Heart, Training the Brain, by America Bracho, Ginger Lee, Gloria P. Goraldo and Rosa María De Prado, tells the story of how Latino Health Access developed its groundbreaking model of peer-to-peer outreach and education in Santa Ana, California to address health problems exacerbated by poverty and discrimination. Their strategies and accomplishments will inspire change across an increasingly unhealthy America. 288 pages.

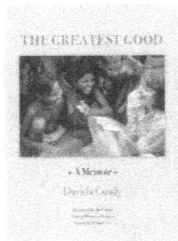

The Greatest Good, a memoir by Dr. Davida Coady, recounts an adventurous life in international public health. From Biafra to Bangladesh, Ethiopia to El Salvador, smallpox eradication to drug rehabilitation, Dr. Coady relates an inspirational life richly and well-lived, driven by the motto: The Greatest Good for the Greatest Number of People. 396 pages.

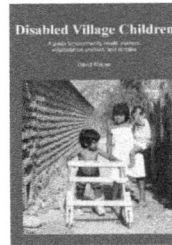

Disabled Village Children, by David Werner, covers most common disabilities of children, giving suggestions for rehabilitation and explaining how to make a variety of low-cost aids. Emphasis is placed on how to help children with disabilities find a role and be accepted in the community. 672 pages.

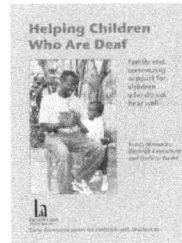

Helping Children Who Are Deaf, by Darlena David, Devorah Greenstein and Sandy Niemann, aids parents, teachers, and other caregivers to help deaf children learn basic communications skills and language. Includes simple methods to assess hearing, develop listening skills, and explore community support for deaf children. 256 pages.

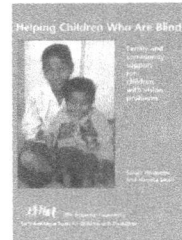

Helping Children Who Are Blind, by Sandy Niemann and Namita Jacob, aids parents and caregivers of blind children from birth to age 5 develop all their capabilities. Topics include: assessing how much a child can see, preventing blindness, moving around safely, teaching common activities, and many others. 200 pages.

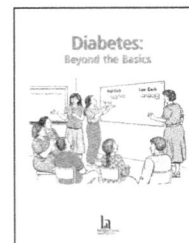

Diabetes: Beyond the Basics is for people living with diabetes, family members, and health workers. This 40-page booklet addresses the physical and social issues of diabetes, and provides discussion questions for health educators and self-help groups.

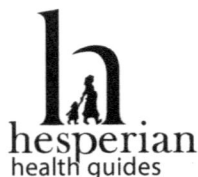

hesperian
health guides
2860 Telegraph Avenue
Oakland, CA 94609 USA

All our books are available in multiple languages.
See www.hesperian.org for details.

To purchase books:
tel: (510) 845-4507
email: bookorders@hesperian.org
online: store.hesperian.org

Distance Vision Acuity Chart — for use at 3 meters (10 feet)

This box should measure 2cm x 2cm

20/200	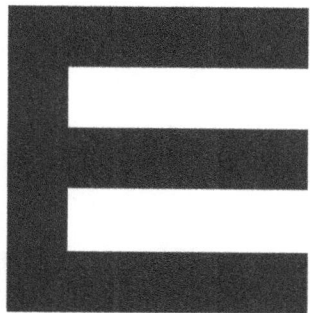	6/60
20/120	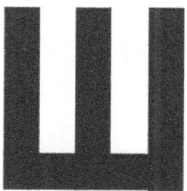	6/36
20/80	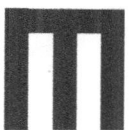	6/24
20/60		6/18
20/40		6/12
20/30		6/9
20/20		6/6

Adapted from Matthew Smith, 2009, by Hesperian Health Guides

hesperian health guides

www.ingramcontent.com/pod-product-compliance
Lightning Source LLC
Chambersburg PA
CBHW081724290326
41933CB00053B/3360